SPINAL CORD INJURY NATURAL REMEDY BOOK

A DETAILED RECOVERY GUIDE FROM PAIN TO SOUND HEALTH

CELIA NELSON

AMAZON

CONTENTS

CHAPTER 1

UNDERSTANDING SPINAL CORD INJURIES

Anatomy of Spinal Cord

The spinal cord is a long, thin, tubular structure composed of neural tissue that runs from the brainstem to the lower back. It is encased within the vertebral column (spine) and comprises the following essential components:

Vertebrae are the bones that make up the spine and provide structural support and protection to the spinal cord.

Nerves are bundles of nerve fibres that carry signals between the brain and the rest of the body.

The spinal cord is divided into five segments: cervical, thoracic, lumbar, sacral, and coccygeal. Each section represents a specific body area or function.

Types of Spinal Cord Injuries:

Spinal cord injuries (SCI) are classed according to the severity and location of the injury.

Complete Injury: Loss of all motor and sensory function below the level of injury.

Incomplete Injury: Partial loss of function occurs when some motor or sensory function persists below the injury level.

Injuries can also be classified according to the spinal cord section affected.

Cervical (neck): May cause quadriplegia or tetraplegia (loss of function in the arms, legs, and torso).

Thoracic (upper back): Can result in paraplegia (loss of function in the lower body).

Lumbar (lower back): Frequently impairs leg and lower body functions.

Sacral (pelvic): Generally affects the hips, thighs, and pelvic organs.

Causes and Risk Factors

Spinal cord injuries can occur from a variety of traumatic and non-traumatic events:

Traumatic Causes:

Motor vehicle accidents are a leading cause, particularly among young individuals.

Falls are common among older persons.

Sports Injuries: Especially in contact and intense sports.

Violence: This includes gunshot wounds and stabbings.

Diving accidents: Caused by shallow water hits.

Non-Traumatic Causes:

Diseases include cancer, arthritis, and osteoporosis.

Infections include meningitis and abscesses.

Degenerative conditions include spinal stenosis.

Risk factors for SCI include age, gender (males have a higher prevalence), and participation in high-risk activities.

Symptoms and diagnoses

The symptoms of spinal cord injuries vary depending on the severity and location:

Motor Function Loss: Weakness or paralysis in the limbs.

Sensory function loss includes numbness, tingling, and loss of sensation.

Autonomic function disruption includes problems with bowel and bladder control, blood pressure, and respiration.

Pain: Persistent discomfort at or below the injury site.

The diagnosis of SCI consists of multiple steps:

The initial assessment involves evaluating motor and sensory function, reflexes, and respiration.

Imaging studies include X-rays, MRIs, and CT scans to help determine the amount and location of the injury.

A neurological examination is performed by a specialist to determine the severity and extent of the injury.

Early and correct diagnosis is crucial for developing an effective treatment plan and improving the prognosis.

CHAPTER 2

THE SCIENCE OF NATURAL REMEDIES

Natural healing is the use of non-invasive, holistic ways to stimulate the body's own healing mechanisms. This method treats the entire person—mind, body, and spirit—rather than just the symptoms.

The holistic approach integrates physical, emotional, mental, and spiritual wellbeing. It emphasises the body's natural potential to repair itself when given the proper conditions and assistance.

Whole-Person Care: Treatments are personalised to each individual in order to restore balance and improve overall well-being.

Natural remedies

Natural remedies refer to a variety of therapies and substances originating from nature, such as herbs, foods, and physical routines.

Focus: These treatments are intended to assist the body's natural functioning and promote recovery without the use of synthetic medications or invasive procedures.

Benefits and Limitations

Natural medicines provide a number of benefits, but they also have limitations.

Benefits

Natural medicines tend to have fewer and milder side effects than pharmaceutical drugs.

Holistic Wellness: They frequently promote overall health and well-being by addressing several elements of health at once.

Cost-effectiveness: Many natural medicines are inexpensive and easily accessible.

Empowerment: Patients frequently feel more in control of their health when they can actively participate in their therapy.

Limitations

Variable Effectiveness: The efficacy of natural therapies might differ greatly between individuals.

Lack of Regulation: Certain natural goods are not carefully controlled, resulting in variances in quality and purity.

Scientific Evidence: While many natural medicines have a long history of use, others lack rigorous scientific research to back up their efficacy.

Not a Cure-All: Natural remedies may not be effective as single treatments for serious diseases and should be combined with conventional therapy.

Integrating Natural Remedies and Conventional Treatments

Combining natural therapies with conventional medicines can improve treatment outcomes and patient well-being.

Alternative care

Synergy: Natural medicines can supplement conventional treatments by reducing adverse effects, strengthening the immune system, and hastening recovery.

Holistic Benefits: Natural remedies can assist manage chronic diseases and enhance overall quality of life.

Communication with healthcare providers.

Transparency is essential for informing healthcare practitioners about all natural medicines utilised to avoid potential interactions with conventional treatments.

Collaborative Care: Working with healthcare experts to develop an integrated treatment plan ensures that all elements of health are treated safely and effectively.

Scientific Basis of Natural Remedies

Understanding the scientific basis of natural medicines allows you to appreciate their potential benefits as well as their limitations.

Phytotherapy, often known as herbal medicine, involves using plant-based medicines to treat various illnesses. Many herbs include bioactive chemicals with medicinal benefits, such as anti-inflammatory, antioxidant, and analgesic qualities.

Nutritional Science

Diet and Health: Proper nutrition is essential for overall health. Vitamins, minerals, and antioxidants are essential for cellular repair, immunological function, and overall health.

Functional foods include probiotics, omega-3 fatty acids, and fibre, which provide health advantages in addition to basic nutrition.

Mind/Body Medicine

Psychoneuroimmunology is the study of how psychological processes interact with the neurological and immune systems. Meditation and mindfulness techniques can help to regulate stress and promote healing.

Neuroplasticity is the brain's ability to reorganise itself by creating new neural connections. Meditation and visualisation are two practices that can improve neuroplasticity and help people heal from injuries.

Physical therapies

Biomechanics is the study of the motion and mechanics of the human body. Yoga, pilates, and hydrotherapy all help to enhance strength, flexibility, and functional movement.

Pain Management: Natural therapies such as acupuncture, chiropractic care, and massage therapy help to manage pain by altering the nerve system and increasing circulation.

Evidence-based Natural Remedies

Several natural therapies have been investigated and supported by scientific investigation.

Omega 3 Fatty Acids

Source: Fish oil and flaxseed.

Benefits include anti-inflammatory qualities that alleviate pain and promote nerve health.

Curcumin (turmeric)

Source: Turmeric contains an active chemical.

Benefits include strong anti-inflammatory and antioxidant properties. Research backs up its usage in lowering pain and inflammation in a variety of illnesses.

Meditation & Mindfulness

Numerous studies have found that these behaviours reduce stress, improve mental health, and boost general well-being.

Mechanisms: Affect brain function, lower cortisol levels, and increase emotional control.

Acupuncture

Research has shown that it is useful for pain management, inflammatory reduction, and general health improvement.

Mechanisms: Stimulates certain spots on the body to regulate nervous system activity and promote healing.

The evidence underpinning natural therapies supports their use as effective and complementary treatments for a wide range of diseases, including spinal cord injury. While they provide several benefits, it is critical to approach them with an understanding of their limitations and to carefully combine them with traditional medical care for the best health outcomes.

CHAPTER 3

Nutrition and Diet

Developing a food plan for someone with a spinal cord injury entails focusing on nutrients that promote overall health, reduce inflammation, and aid in healing and nerve function. Here's a complete eating plan suited to the needs of people with spinal cord injuries:

The Best Diet Plan for Spinal Cord Injury

Key Nutritional Goals

Reduce Inflammation: Anti-inflammatory foods can help control chronic pain and inflammation.

Promote Healing: Provide nutrients required for tissue repair and nerve health.

Prevent Complications: Address any potential difficulties such as constipation, pressure sores, and weight control.

Boost the Immune System: Improve general health and resistance to infection.

Daily Meal Plan: Breakfast

Green Smoothie: Combine spinach, kale, banana, berries (blueberries and strawberries), chia seeds, and almond milk.

Benefits: Rich in antioxidants, vitamins, and fibre, which promote immunological health and digestion.

Whole Grain Toast with Avocado: Sprinkle with chia or flaxseed.

Benefits include healthy fats, fibre, and omega-3 fatty acids, which help to reduce inflammation and promote heart health.

Greek Yoghurt: Combine plain Greek yoghurt with walnuts and honey.

Benefits include probiotics for digestive health, protein for muscle maintenance, and omega-3s from walnuts.

Mid-morning snack

Apple Slices with Almond Butter: A sliced apple with a scoop of almond butter.

Benefits include fibre, healthy fats, and antioxidants.

Lunch

Grilled Salmon Salad includes mixed greens, cherry tomatoes, cucumbers, carrots, and grilled salmon. Drizzle with olive oil and lemon juice.

Omega-3 fatty acids have anti-inflammatory properties, whereas protein aids in tissue regeneration.

Quinoa or brown rice: A small dish on the side.

Benefits include complex carbohydrates for sustained energy and fibre.

Afternoon Snack

Hummus & Veggie Sticks: Carrots, celery, bell peppers, and hummus.

Benefits include fibre, vitamins, and protein.

Dinner

Baked chicken breast seasoned with herbs and spices, served with steamed broccoli and sweet potato.

Benefits include lean protein for muscular maintenance and micronutrients from vegetables.

Mixed Vegetable Stir-fry: Cook bell peppers, zucchini, mushrooms, and snap peas in olive oil with garlic and ginger.

Benefits: Rich in antioxidants, vitamins, and anti-inflammatory substances.

Evening Snack.

Chia Pudding: Soak chia seeds in almond milk overnight and top with fresh berries.

Benefits include omega-3 fatty acids, fibre, and antioxidants.

Nutritional Supplements

Omega-3 Fatty Acids: Supplements including fish oil or flaxseed oil might help reduce inflammation.

Vitamin D is essential for bone health, especially if mobility is restricted.

Vitamin B12 promotes nerve health and energy levels.

Probiotics: To keep your gut healthy and prevent constipation.

Magnesium: Improves muscle function and can relieve cramps and spasms.

Drink at least 8 glasses of water daily to maintain hydration and support body processes.

Herbal teas such as green tea, chamomile, and peppermint can help with relaxation while also providing antioxidants.

Additional Tips:

Fibre Intake: To avoid constipation, consume an adequate amount of fibre. Incorporate entire grains, fruits, veggies, and legumes.

Avocados, almonds, seeds, and olive oil are good sources of healthy fats, which can help with brain and nerve function.

Protein: Include lean protein sources in each meal to aid in muscle maintenance and regeneration.

Meal Timing: Eat smaller, more frequent meals to retain energy and avoid blood sugar rises.

Individuals with spinal cord injuries can promote their body's healing processes, reduce inflammation, and improve general health and well-being by eating a balanced and nutrient-dense diet.

CHAPTER 4

Physical Therapies

Physical therapy are critical components of the recovery process for people with spinal cord injuries (SCI). These therapies are intended to preserve and improve physical function, mobility, and overall quality of life. Here's a detailed look at the numerous physical therapy that can help SCI patients:

Yoga and Stretching Exercises

Yoga and stretching exercises can dramatically improve the flexibility, strength, and mental health of those with SCI.

Benefits

Regular stretching helps to maintain and increase range of motion.

Strengthens Muscles: Certain yoga positions work on muscles, especially the core.

Improves Mental Health: Yoga promotes relaxation while lowering stress, anxiety, and depression.

Pain Relief: Gentle stretching might help with muscle stiffness and chronic pain.

Specific poses and exercises

Seated Forward Bend stretches the spine, shoulders, and hamstrings.

Cat-Cow Stretch: Increases spinal flexibility and warms the spine.

Seated Twist improves spinal mobility and digestion.

Wheelchair Yoga: Adapted poses for wheelchair users to increase flexibility and strength without leaving their chair.

Pilates for Core Strengthening

Pilates emphasises core strength, stability, and controlled movements, all of which are essential for SCI therapy.

Focus and Benefits

Core Strength: Strong core muscles help to support the spine while also improving balance and posture.

Pilates workouts improve coordination and general body stability.

Low Impact: Because the movements are controlled and moderate, they are appropriate for anyone with restricted mobility.

Spinal Support: Assists in preserving spinal alignment and relieving discomfort.

Key Exercises

Pelvic tilts help to strengthen the lower abdominal muscles and enhance pelvic stability.

Leg Slides: Engage the core muscles while allowing for modest leg movement.

Arm and Leg Reach: Enhances balance and coordination while strengthening core muscles.

Modified Planks: Strengthens the shoulders, arms, and core with adjustments for different levels of mobility.

Hydrotherapy

Hydrotherapy, also known as aquatic therapy, consists of water activities that provide a supportive and low-impact environment for rehabilitation.

Advantages

Buoyancy: Water supports the body, relieving pressure on muscles and joints.

Resistance: Water resistance strengthens muscles while reducing the chance of damage.

Warm water can help relieve discomfort and relax tense muscles.

Improved Circulation: Hydrotherapy increases blood flow, which aids healing and reduces edema.

Types of Exercise

Walking in water helps to increase leg strength and balance.

Leg Lifts: Using water resistance to strengthen the legs and core.

Arm exercises involve pushing and pulling actions in water to increase upper body strength.

Floating and Stretching: Use water's buoyancy to gently stretch muscles.

Acupuncture and acupressure

Acupuncture and acupressure stimulate specific areas on the body to promote healing and alleviate pain.

Mechanism

Acupuncture is the insertion of tiny needles into particular locations to stimulate the nervous system and encourage the release of endorphins.

Acupressure: Applying pressure to these spots with hands, elbows, or devices to elicit comparable results.

Benefits

Pain Relief: Effective for alleviating chronic pain and muscular spasms.

Improved Circulation: Increases blood flow to wounded areas, which promotes healing.

Stress Reduction: Reduces stress and anxiety, promoting general well-being.

Improved Mobility: Promotes range of motion and reduces stiffness.

Common Points for SCI

GV (Governing Vessel) Points: Along the spine, beneficial to spinal health.

BL (Bladder) Points: Found near the spinal column, they help with pain alleviation and mobility.

Additional Physical Therapies.

Aside from the basic therapies outlined above, other physical therapies can play a key role in SCI rehabilitation:

Occupational Therapy

Focuses on assisting patients in performing everyday activities independently.

Includes instruction on the use of adapted equipment and strategies to improve functionality and quality of life.

Electrical Stimulation

Stimulates nerves and muscles with electrical currents.

Helps to preserve muscular mass, reduce stiffness, and improve motor function.

Massage Therapy

Muscles and soft tissues are manipulated manually.

Reduces muscle tension, boosts circulation, and encourages relaxation.

Physical Therapy

Aims to restore movement and function through personalised exercise programmes.

Strength training, balancing exercises, and gait training are provided for individuals who can walk.

Creating a personalised physical therapy plan

Developing a personalised physical therapy plan is critical for successful rehabilitation and recovery. Here are the important steps for creating such a plan:

Initial Assessment

Assess the patient's present physical condition, mobility, and specific needs.

Determine therapy objectives, such as improving mobility, relieving pain, or increasing independence.

Tailored Exercise Programme

Create an exercise programme tailored to the patient's ability and goals.

Include a variety of strength, stretching, and cardio workouts.

Regular Monitoring and Adjustments

Monitor the patient's progress on a frequent basis.

Adjust the therapy plan as necessary based on progress and any changes in condition.

Integration of Other Therapies

Combine physical therapies with other treatments such as medication, nutritional support, and mental health counselling.

Maintain a holistic approach to healing.

Patient Education and Involvement

Educate the patient on the value of consistency and adherence to the treatment plan.

Encourage active engagement and self-management for the condition.

CHAPTER 5

Mind-Body Techniques

Mind-body approaches are therapies that emphasise the interplay of the mind and body in order to improve physical, mental, and emotional well-being. These strategies can be especially effective for people with spinal cord injuries (SCI) since they assist control pain, reduce stress, and enhance overall quality of life.

Meditation and Mindfulness Practices

Mindfulness meditation involves paying attention to the current moment without judgement. This technique can assist SCI patients cope with stress and suffering by developing a non-reactive awareness of their circumstances.

Guided Imagery is a technique that uses visualisation to aid relaxation and healing. Patients picture calm images or hopeful outcomes to alleviate stress and improve mental health.

Loving-Kindness Meditation focuses on developing compassion and love for oneself and others, which helps boost mental health and resilience.

Benefits

Reduces Stress and Anxiety: Mindfulness and meditation reduce the body's stress response by reducing cortisol and other stress hormones.

Improves Pain Management: By diverting the emphasis away from pain and encouraging a sense of calm, these activities can lower pain perception.

Improves Mental Health: Regular practice helps reduce symptoms of depression and anxiety, fostering a cheerful attitude.

Breathing Exercises and Techniques

Diaphragmatic breathing refers to deep breathing from the diaphragm rather than shallow breathing from the chest. This approach improves oxygenation and encourages relaxation.

Paced breathing is the process of regulating one's breathing rate, usually by counting or following a set beat. Helps to manage anxiety and reduce the stress reaction.

Alternate Nostril Breathing is a yoga technique in which one breathes through each nostril alternately. This exercise is thought to help regulate the nervous system and increase mental clarity.

Impact

Deep, controlled breathing activates the parasympathetic nervous system, leading to a sense of calm.

Reduces Pain: Better oxygenation and relaxation help to manage pain levels.

Improves Focus: Controlled breathing can help you concentrate and think clearly.

Biofeedback Process

Monitoring: Biofeedback employs electronic equipment to track physiological functions such as heart rate, muscle tension, and body temperature.

Patients get real-time feedback on their physiological states, which helps them learn how to control these processes consciously.

Training: Patients gradually learn to control their physiological responses to stress, pain, and other stimuli.

Applications

Pain Management: Assists patients in relieving muscle tension and managing chronic pain more effectively.

Stress Reduction: teaches patients how to control their stress responses, which leads to less anxiety and more relaxation.

Improved Function: Can help you regain control of specific physiological functions that may be impaired by SCI.

Visualisation and Guided Imagery Methods

Healing Imagery: Patients visualise their spinal cord being healed and their bodily functions improving.

Relaxation Imagery: Visualising pleasant and serene settings to relieve stress and promote relaxation.

Goal-Oriented Imagery: Visualising the successful completion of specified tasks, such as walking or performing an activity.

Uses

Pain Management: Visualisation helps lower pain perception by diverting attention and instilling a sense of control.

Stress Reduction: Imagery promotes relaxation and reduces stress by immersing the mind in happy and relaxing settings.

Enhanced Recovery: Positive imagery can increase motivation and encourage a proactive approach to rehabilitation.

Cognitive Behavioural Therapy (CBT) Principles

Cognitive restructuring involves identifying and confronting problematic thought patterns in order to replace them with positive, adaptive ones.

Behavioural activation is encouraging participation in activities that provide a sense of accomplishment and delight, which improves mood and motivation.

Techniques

Thought Records: Keeping track of negative ideas and assessing their validity.

Activity scheduling entails planning and participating in fun and meaningful activities to combat depression and increase quality of life.

The effects

Improves Mental Health: Helps to reduce symptoms of depression and anxiety.

Improves Coping Skills: Assists patients in developing healthier methods to cope with the problems of SCI.

Promotes Positive Thinking: Encourages a proactive approach to rehabilitation.

Integrating Mind-Body Techniques.

Holistic Approach

Combination Therapies: Combining several mind-body techniques can improve their overall effectiveness. Meditation, for example, can be practised in addition to visualisation and breathing exercises.

Personalisation: Tailoring tactics to individual preferences and needs leads to higher engagement and outcomes.

Regular Practice: Consistency is essential for receiving the benefits of mind-body methods. Establishing a consistent schedule aids in the integration of these activities into daily life.

Communication with healthcare providers.

Informed Choices: Patients should consult with their healthcare practitioners before using mind-body therapies to ensure they complement the entire treatment plan.

Monitoring Progress: Regular monitoring and input from healthcare practitioners might assist in altering strategies to maximise benefit.

Support and Resources

Professional Guidance: Working with skilled specialists such as psychologists, therapists, or certified instructors can help these strategies work more effectively.

CHAPTER 6

ALTERNATIVE AND COMPLEMENTARY THERAPIES

Alternative and complementary therapies refer to a wide range of treatments that are used in conjunction with or instead of traditional medical treatments. These therapies can help people with spinal cord injuries (SCI) manage their pain, enhance their mobility, and feel better overall.

Alternative Therapies: Treatments that replace conventional medicine.

Complementary Therapies: therapies used in conjunction with conventional medical therapies to increase their efficacy and patient outcomes.

Goals

Pain Management: Reducing the chronic pain and suffering caused by SCI.

Improved Mobility: Increases physical function and range of motion.

Mental and Emotional Support: Addressing the psychological effects of SCI.

Holistic Well-Being: Improving overall health and quality of life.

Acupuncture principles

Traditional Chinese Medicine (TCM): Acupuncture works by balancing the body's energy flow (Qi) through specific places on the body known as acupoints.

Needle Insertion: Fine needles are introduced into the skin at appropriate locations to activate nerves, muscles, and connective tissues.

Benefits

Pain Relief: Effective at alleviating chronic pain, muscle spasms, and neuropathic pain.

Improved Circulation: Increases blood flow, promotes healing, and decreases inflammation.

Stress Reduction: Helps to relieve stress, anxiety, and sadness.

Application

Pain Management: Acupuncture can be used to treat pain in a variety of areas of the body, including the back, neck, and legs.

Functional Improvement: Can help to improve motor function and movement.

Chiropractic Care Principles

Spinal Manipulation: Chiropractic therapy includes physical adjustments to the spine and other joints to enhance alignment and function.

Holistic Approach: Emphasises the connection between the spine and the neural system, supporting total wellness.

Benefits

Pain Reduction: Effective for relieving back pain, neck discomfort, and headaches.

Improved Mobility: Improves joint mobility and flexibility.

Nervous System Support: Helps to keep the nervous system healthy.

Application

Spinal Adjustments: These are regular adjustments made to rectify spinal misalignments.

Exercise and Rehabilitation: Uses exercises and stretches to aid in rehabilitation and preserve health.

Herbal Medicine Principles.

Natural Remedies: Uses plant-based ingredients to treat a variety of ailments and promote health.

Traditional Knowledge: Based on traditional therapeutic practices and knowledge of medicinal herbs.

Common Herbs for SCI.

Turmeric (Curcumin) contains anti-inflammatory and

antioxidant qualities that can help alleviate pain and inflammation.

Ginger contains anti-inflammatory and pain-relieving qualities.

Ginkgo Biloba: May boost circulation and neurological health.

Valerian root is used for its soothing properties and pain treatment.

Benefits

Natural Pain Relief: Offers alternative pain management methods without the side effects associated with pharmaceutical medicines.

Anti-Inflammatory: Decreases inflammation and promotes healing.

Holistic Health: Enhances overall well-being.

Massage Therapy Principles

Manual Manipulation is the manipulation of muscles, tendons, and other soft tissues to release tension and induce relaxation.

Various Techniques: Includes Swedish massage, deep tissue massage, trigger point therapy, and other treatments.

Benefits

Pain Relief: Lowers muscle tension and relieves pain.

Improved Circulation: Increases blood flow and promotes healing.

Relaxation alleviates stress and anxiety, hence boosting mental health.

Application

Targeted Therapy: Concentrates on the areas afflicted by SCI to alleviate specific symptoms.

Regular massage therapy sessions can provide long-term advantages and aid with rehabilitation.

Reiki & Energy Healing Principles

Energy Balance: Reiki is founded on the concept of life force energy and seeks to balance it inside the body.

Non-invasive: Uses light touch or hovering hands over the body to direct healing energy.

Benefits

Stress Reduction: Encourages deep relaxation and relieves stress.

Pain Management: Can help to relieve pain and discomfort.

Emotional healing promotes emotional well-being and lowers anxiety.

Application

Reiki treatments are regular sessions with a qualified practitioner that promote healing and balance.

Self-Practice: Patients can learn simple self-care practices.

Aromatherapy Principles

Essential oils are concentrated plant extracts used for medicinal purposes.

Inhalation or topical application: Oils can be breathed or

massaged into the skin.

Benefits

Pain Relief: Essential oils such as lavender and eucalyptus have pain-relieving effects.

Stress Reduction: Oils such as lavender, chamomile, and bergamot help to relax and reduce anxiety.

Aromatherapy can boost mood and emotional well-being.

Application

Diffusers: Using diffusers to disseminate essential oils into the air.

Massage: Adding essential oils to massage therapy for additional advantages.

Topical Use: Applying diluted essential oils to the skin to achieve certain effects.

Integrative Approach - Combining Therapies

Synergy: Combining several therapies can improve overall effectiveness while also addressing multiple health concerns.

Personalisation involves tailoring the combination of therapies to the individual's needs, preferences, and response.

Collaborating with healthcare providers to develop integrated care programmes that include traditional and alternative therapies.

Monitoring and Adjustment: The therapy plan is regularly monitored and adjusted to get the best possible outcomes.

Patient Education and Involvement

Enlightened Choices: Providing patients with information about the benefits and limitations of various therapy so that they can make informed decisions.

Active Participation: Encouraging patients to actively participate in their recovery and treatment.

CHAPTER 7

LIFESTYLE MODIFICATIONS

Individuals with spinal cord injuries (SCI) benefit greatly from lifestyle adjustments. These adjustments can help with symptom management, preventing problems, and improving quality of life. Here's a detailed look at numerous lifestyle alterations that benefit SCI patients:

Physical Activity and Exercise: Why It Matters

Maintains Muscle Strength: Prevents muscle atrophy and keeps muscles toned.

Improves Cardiovascular Health: Lowers the risk of cardiovascular problems, which are prevalent in those with limited mobility.

Improves Mood and Mental Health: Physical activity produces endorphins, which improve mood and alleviate symptoms of despair and anxiety.

Types of Exercise

Strength training focuses on maintaining and increasing muscle strength. Use resistance bands, weights, or bodyweight workouts.

Cardiovascular Exercise: Swimming, stationary bike riding, and hand cycling can all help to enhance cardiovascular health.

Stretching and yoga increase flexibility, reduce muscular stiffness, and improve range of motion.

Functional training involves exercises that simulate daily activities in order to increase functional abilities and independence.

Adaptations and Assistive Devices

Wheelchair-Accessible Equipment: Many gyms have equipment specifically built for wheelchair users, such as hand cycles and accessible weight machines.

Home Exercise Programmes: Customised exercises that may be completed at home with little equipment.

Physical Therapy: Collaborating with a physical therapist to create a safe and effective exercise programme.

Nutrition and Diet Goals:

Support Healing and Recovery: Nutrients that promote tissue repair and minimise inflammation.

Weight Management: Avoid weight gain due to limited movement, which might lead to extra health problems.

Improve Digestive Health: Address frequent concerns such as constipation in SCI patients.

Key Nutrients

Protein is essential for muscle repair and rehabilitation. Incorporate lean meats, fish, eggs, beans, and dairy.

Fibre promotes digestion and reduces constipation. Fruits, vegetables, whole grains, and legumes are all potential sources.

Healthy Fats: Omega-3 fatty acids lower inflammation and promote brain health. Found in fish, flaxseeds, chia seeds, and walnuts.

Vitamins and Minerals: Ensure a proper intake of vitamins and minerals, particularly vitamin D and calcium, for bone health.

Dietary Tips:

A balanced diet should include a range of nutrients.

Hydration: Drink enough water to stay hydrated and promote good health.

Meal Planning: Plan meals and snacks to meet nutritional requirements and avoid harmful eating habits.

Mental and emotional health challenges.

Depression and anxiety are common in people with SCI owing to changes in their lifestyle and mobility.

Adjustment issues include adjusting to a new way of life and dealing with the obstacles that come with it.

Support Strategies

Therapy and Counselling: Attending regular appointments with a psychologist or counsellor might help you manage your mental health.

Help Groups: Connecting with others who have gone through similar circumstances can provide emotional and practical help.

Meditation, mindfulness, and relaxation activities can help to reduce stress and enhance mental health.

Participation in Activities: Engaging in hobbies and social activities to preserve a sense of meaning and satisfaction.

Environmental adaptations

Home Modifications

Accessibility: Make sure the home environment is wheelchair accessible. This includes ramps, wide doorways, and accessible restrooms and kitchens.

Assistive gadgets: Use of gadgets such as grab bars, transfer benches, and adaptable kitchenware to increase independence.

Workplace Adaptations

Reasonable Accommodations: Changes in the work environment or schedule to accommodate mobility restrictions.

Ergonomic Workstations: Creating a workspace that minimises strain and increases comfort.

Transportation

Accessible automobiles: Use wheelchair-accessible automobiles or public transportation choices developed specifically for people with impairments.

Travel Planning: Making advance plans to ensure accessibility while travelling, such as lodging, transportation, and activities.

Prevention of Secondary Complications

Pressure ulcers

Changing positions regularly to alleviate pressure.

Specialised Cushions and Mattresses: Use pressure-relieving cushions and mattresses to avoid skin deterioration.

Skin care entails keeping the skin clean and moisturise while also checking it on a regular basis for symptoms of pressure sores.

Urinary Tract Infections (UTI)

Hydration entails drinking plenty of fluids to flush out the urinary system.

Catheter Care: To avoid infections, maintain proper cleanliness and change catheters on a regular basis.

Regular monitoring involves being aware of symptoms and seeking timely treatment for UTIs.

Osteoporosis, Bone Health

Weight-Bearing Exercises: If possible, participate in weight-bearing exercises to strengthen your bones.

Calcium and Vitamin D: Ensure that you get enough calcium and vitamin D to maintain your bones.

Respiratory Health

Breathing Exercises: Techniques for strengthening respiratory muscles and improving lung function.

CHAPTER 8

Herbal Remedies

Herbal treatments have been used for years to treat a range of disorders, and they can provide numerous benefits to people who have suffered spinal cord injuries (SCI). These natural remedies can help manage pain, reduce inflammation, promote healing, and boost overall health. This is a complete guide on using herbal medicines for SCI.

What are Herbal Remedies?

Herbal medicines are treatments made from plants and their extracts, such as leaves, roots, bark, flowers, and seeds.

Forms include teas, tinctures, capsules, powders, and topical treatments.

Principles of Herbal Medicine

Herbal medicines use a holistic approach, treating the entire individual rather than simply symptoms.

Inherent Healing: Uses the body's inherent healing processes to promote balance and wellness.

Common Herbal Remedies for SCI: Anti-inflammatory Herbs

Turmeric (Curcumin) offers powerful anti-inflammatory and antioxidant effects.

Usage: It can be taken as a supplement, in food, or in tea.

Mechanism: It reduces inflammation by blocking specific molecules involved in the inflammatory process.

Ginger reduces inflammation and pain.

Fresh ginger can be added to cuisine, brewed into tea, or taken as a supplement.

Mechanism: Contains chemicals with anti-inflammatory and analgesic properties, such as gingerol.

Pain-relieving herbs

Willow Bark

Benefits: Natural pain reliever, often known as "nature's aspirin."

Available in tea, pill, and tincture form.

Mechanism: Salicin is converted by the body into salicylic acid, which reduces pain and inflammation.

Devil's Claw

Benefits: Effective in relieving pain, especially in the lower back.

Usage: Usually taken in capsule or tincture form.

Mechanism: Harpagoside contains anti-inflammatory and analgesic effects.

Nerve Health and Repair Herbs

St. John's Wort promotes nerve health and lowers neuropathic pain.

Usage options include tea, oil, and supplements.

Mechanism: It contains hypericin and hyperforin, which may aid in nerve repair and function.

Ginkgo Biloba

Benefits: Promotes circulation and nerve health.

Usage options include tea, extract, and capsules.

Mechanism: Increases blood flow to the neurological system and gives antioxidant protection.

Herbs for Muscle spasms and relaxation

Valerian root benefits include natural muscle relaxation and sedation.

Available in tea, tincture, and pill form.

Mechanism: Increases gamma-aminobutyric acid (GABA) levels in the brain, which promotes relaxation.

Chamomile

Benefits: Reduces muscle spasms and encourages relaxation.

Usage: Typically drunk as tea.

Mechanism: Flavonoids with antispasmodic and sedative properties.

Herbs For Digestive Health

Peppermint

Benefits: Reduces digestive problems including bloating and cramps.

Consumption options include tea, oil, and capsules.

Mechanism: Menthol relaxes the muscles of the gastrointestinal tract.

Slippery Elm

Benefits: It soothes the digestive tract and relieves constipation.

Usage: Available as a powder to combine with water or in capsule form.

Mechanism: mucilage coats and calms the digestive tract.

Herbs for Immune Support.

Echinacea benefits include boosting the immune system and decreasing the frequency of illnesses.

Consume as a tea, tincture, or supplement.

Mechanism: It stimulates the immune system by enhancing the activity of white blood cells.

Astragalus

Benefits: improves immunological function and promotes general health.

Usage options include tea, tincture, and supplement.

Mechanism: Polysaccharides promote immunological activation and healing.

Safety and precautions

Consultation with healthcare providers.

Professional Advice: Always contact a healthcare provider before beginning any herbal therapies, especially if you are using other medications or have pre-existing medical concerns.

Potential Interactions: Some plants can interact with pharmaceuticals, causing side effects.

Quality and Sourcing

Reputable Sources: Buy herbs from reputable vendors to assure quality and purity.

Organic Options: When feasible, use organic herbs to prevent pollutants such as pesticides.

Dosages and Administration

Proper Dosage: To avoid any adverse effects or toxicity, follow the recommended amounts.

Form and Preparation: Learn the optimum form and method of preparation for each plant in order to maximise its effects.

Monitoring and Adjustment

Monitor the effects of the herbal remedies and modify the dosage as needed.

Negative Effects: Be careful of potential negative effects and quit use if any arise.

Adding Herbal Remedies to a Holistic Health Plan

Complementary Approach

Combination with Conventional Treatments: Use herbal medicines as part of a comprehensive treatment plan that includes traditional medical treatments and therapies.

Supportive Therapies: Combine herbal medicines with additional supportive therapies such as physical therapy, diet, and mind-body exercises.

Personalised Treatment Plans

Individual demands: Tailor herbal medicines to the individual's specific demands and situations.

Holistic Approach: When designing a treatment plan, consider all elements of health—physical, mental, and emotional.

CHAPTER 9
Essential Oils

What are Essential Oils?
Definition: Concentrated plant extracts that retain their smell and beneficial characteristics.

Extraction methods: Includes steam or water distillation as well as cold pressing.

Principles of Aromatherapy
Historical Use: Essential oils have been utilised medicinally and therapeutically in diverse civilizations for ages.

Mechanism of Action: The oils can impact the body by inhalation, topical application, interaction with the limbic system in the brain, or skin absorption.

Common Essential Oils for SCI
Pain Relief
Lavender Oil
Benefits include calming, pain-relieving, and anti-inflammatory effects.
Diffusion, topical application (diluted), or immersion in a bath.

Mechanism: Reduces pain by decreasing levels of the neurotransmitter molecule. P. Peppermint Oil.

Benefits include analgesic and cooling effects.
Application: Topical (diluted), inhalation.
Mechanism: Contains menthol, which provides a cooling effect and helps to relieve pain.

Muscle Relaxation
Chamomile Oil

Benefits: It relieves muscle spasms and lowers inflammation.

Application: Topical (diluted) in a bath.

Mechanism: Contains chemicals with anti-inflammatory and muscle-relaxing properties.

Marjoram oil.
Benefits include muscle relaxation and pain relief.
Application: Topical (diluted) and massage.
Mechanism: It has characteristics that assist relax muscles and relieve pain.
Mood Improvement and Stress Reduction

Bergamot Oil
Benefits: Lowers anxiety and boosts happiness.
Usage options include inhalation and topical application (diluted).

Mechanism: Interacts with neurotransmitters to alleviate anxiety and boost mood.

Ylang Ylang Oil.
Benefits: Relaxes the nervous system and reduces anxiety.
Usage options include inhalation and topical application (diluted).
Mechanism: Uses the limbic system to promote relaxation and relieve stress.
Immune Support.

Tea Tree Oil
Benefits include antimicrobial qualities that promote immunological health.

Application: Topical (diluted), inhalation.

Mechanism: Contains chemicals that combat bacteria, viruses, and fungi.

Eucalyptus Oil
Benefits: Improves respiratory health and the immunological system.

Usage options include inhalation and topical application (diluted).

Mechanism: Improves respiratory function and gives antibacterial properties.

Safety and Usage Guidelines

Dilution and Application

To avoid skin irritation, essential oils should be diluted with a carrier oil (such as coconut or jojoba oil) before applying them topically.

Patch Test: Before using a new essential oil, always do a patch test to rule out any allergic reactions.
Methods of Use

To achieve rapid absorption, use a diffuser or inhale directly from the bottle.
Topical Application: Massage diluted oils into the skin, concentrating on areas of pain or tension.

Baths: Add a few drops of essential oil to a warm bath to promote relaxation and pain treatment.
Precautions

Quality: Only use high-quality, pure essential oils from reliable sources.

Contraindications: Some essential oils are not recommended for certain disorders or during pregnancy; see a doctor.

To preserve the effectiveness of essential oils, store them in dark, glass bottles away from direct sunlight.
Supplements and nutraceuticals
Introduction to Supplements and Nutraceuticals.

Definitions
Supplements are oral products containing dietary elements that are designed to supplement a diet.

Nutraceuticals are foods or items that give health and medical benefits, such as illness prevention and therapy.

Role in SCI

Nutritional Support: Supplements and nutraceuticals can assist meet nutritional demands, promote healing, and enhance general health in people with SCI.

Targeted Benefits:
Specific supplements can help with common ailments like inflammation, discomfort, muscle health, and immunological function.

Common Supplements for SCI

Anti-inflammatory and Pain Relief

Omega 3 Fatty Acids

Benefits: Decreases inflammation and promotes nervous system wellness.

Sources: Fish oil supplements and flaxseed oil.

Omega-3s suppress inflammatory pathways and promote cell membrane health.
Curcumin

Benefits include potent anti-inflammatory and antioxidant properties.
Supplements containing turmeric extract.

Mechanism: It reduces inflammation by blocking specific molecules involved in the inflammatory process.

Bone Health.
Calcium
Benefits: Important for bone strength and health.
Calcium supplements and fortified meals are two such sources.

Mechanism: Increases bone density and helps to prevent osteoporosis.
Vitamin D

Benefits: Improves calcium absorption and bone health.
Vitamin D pills and sunshine exposure are two possible sources.

Mechanism: Required for calcium metabolism and bone health.
Nerve Health and Repair

B Vitamins
Benefits: Promotes nerve health and energy generation.
Sources: B-complex supplements.

Mechanism: B vitamins, particularly thiamine, B6 (pyridoxine), and B12 (cobalamin), are essential for nerve function and repair.

Alpha Lipoic Acid.

Benefits: An antioxidant that promotes nerve function and lowers oxidative stress.

Sources: Alpha-lipoic acid supplementation.

Mechanism: lowers oxidative stress and promotes neuron regeneration.
Muscle Health and Spasm

Magnesium

Benefits: Helps to alleviate muscle spasms and improves muscle function.
Magnesium supplements, leafy greens, and nuts are good sources of magnesium.
Mechanism: Required for muscular relaxation and function.
L-Carnitine

Benefits: Promotes muscle health and energy production.
Sources include L-carnitine supplementation, beef, and dairy products.

Mechanism: Transports fatty acids to the mitochondria for energy generation.

Immune Support.

Vitamin C improves immunological function and lowers inflammation.
Sources include vitamin C pills, citrus foods, and berries.

Mechanism: It helps immune cells operate and functions as an antioxidant.

Zinc
Benefits: Improves immunological function and wound healing.

Sources include zinc supplements, pork, and shellfish.

Mechanism: Required for immune cell activity and protein production.